THE COMPLETE HIGH FIBER DIET COOKBOOK FOR BEGINNERS

Eat Your Way to Total Relief from Diverticulitis, Constipation, Hemorrhoids, a Healthier Gut, and Lower Cholesterol

Audrey McAllister, MD

Copyright © 2024 Audrey McAllister, MD

The contents of this publication are protected by copyright law, and all rights are explicitly reserved. Any reproduction, distribution, or transmission of this work in any form or by any means, including photocopying, recording, or electronic methods, without prior written permission from the publisher, is strictly prohibited. The publisher holds the exclusive rights to authorize any such use of the material contained herein.

Exceptions to this restriction may apply in certain circumstances, such as brief quotations used in critical reviews or for other non-commercial purposes permitted by copyright law. However, any such usage must be accompanied by appropriate attribution and citation to the original source.

Requests for permission to use or reproduce any part of this publication should be addressed to the publisher in writing. The publisher reserves the right to grant or deny permission at their discretion, taking into consideration factors such as the intended use, nature of the excerpt, and potential impact on the original work.

Unauthorized reproduction or distribution of copyrighted material is a violation of intellectual property rights and may result in legal consequences. Individuals or entities found to be in breach of copyright law may be subject to legal action, including but not limited to injunctions, damages, and legal fees.

It is the responsibility of all users of this publication to familiarize themselves with and abide by copyright laws and regulations. By accessing or using any part of this work, individuals agree to comply with the terms and conditions set forth by the publisher regarding copyright protection and usage rights.

Table of Contents

FOREWORD

In an age where diet trends come and go, one nutritional element remains consistently championed by health professionals: dietary fiber. The fiber diet, emphasizing the importance of consuming adequate amounts of this essential nutrient, is not just a fleeting trend but a cornerstone of a healthy lifestyle.

Dietary fiber, often simply referred to as fiber, encompasses the indigestible parts of plant foods. Unlike other food components such as fats, proteins, or carbohydrates that your body breaks down and absorbs, fiber passes relatively intact through your stomach, small intestine, and colon, and out of your body. Despite its journey through the digestive system without being absorbed, fiber plays a crucial role in maintaining overall health.

The importance of fiber was first highlighted in the 1970s by Dr. Denis Burkitt, who observed lower rates of certain diseases in African populations with high-fiber diets compared to Western populations. Since then, extensive research has confirmed the myriad health benefits associated with fiber. From improving digestive health to aiding in weight management, reducing cholesterol levels, and controlling blood sugar levels, fiber's contributions to well-being are extensive and well-documented.

A fiber-rich diet focuses on the consumption of whole, plant-based foods such as fruits, vegetables, whole grains, legumes, nuts, and seeds. These foods are not only high in fiber but also packed with essential vitamins, minerals, and antioxidants, making them invaluable components of a balanced diet.

We will explore the many facets of the fiber diet. You will learn about the different types of fiber, their sources, and how they affect your body. We will delve into the health benefits of a high-fiber diet, provide practical tips for incorporating more fiber into your daily meals, and address common challenges you might face along the way.

Whether you are looking to improve your digestive health, manage your weight, or simply adopt a healthier lifestyle, the fiber diet offers a sustainable and effective approach. By understanding and embracing the principles of the fiber diet, you can take a significant step towards achieving and maintaining optimal health.

Join us as we embark on this journey to uncover the power of fiber and discover how it can transform your health, one meal at a time.

SECTION 1: What is the Fiber Diet?

The Fiber Diet is a comprehensive nutritional approach designed to increase the intake of dietary fiber from a variety of whole, natural foods, including fruits, vegetables, whole grains, legumes, nuts, and seeds. The primary objective of this diet is to leverage the numerous health benefits associated with a high-fiber intake. These benefits include improved digestive health, better weight management, and a reduced risk of chronic diseases such as cardiovascular disease, type 2 diabetes, and certain types of cancer.

A key aspect of the Fiber Diet is its focus on consuming both soluble and insoluble fibers, which play different roles in the body. Soluble fiber dissolves in water to form a gel-like substance that can help lower blood cholesterol and glucose levels.

It is found in foods like oats, peas, beans, apples, citrus fruits, carrots, barley, and psyllium. Insoluble fiber, on the other hand, promotes the movement of material through the digestive system and increases stool bulk, aiding those who struggle with constipation or irregular stools. This type of fiber is found in foods such as whole wheat flour, wheat bran, nuts, beans, and vegetables like cauliflower, green beans, and potatoes.

The Fiber Diet encourages the consumption of fiber-rich foods throughout the day, integrating them into every meal and snack. This approach not only helps in maintaining consistent energy levels and preventing overeating by promoting a feeling of fullness but also ensures a steady supply of essential vitamins, minerals, and other nutrients that support overall health.

The Fiber Diet emphasizes gradual changes in dietary habits to prevent digestive discomfort that can arise from a sudden increase in fiber intake. It advocates for a balanced diet that includes adequate hydration, as water is essential for fiber to work effectively in the digestive system.

A High Fiber Diet is not just a temporary dietary plan but a sustainable lifestyle change aimed at improving long-term health outcomes. By fostering a diet rich in natural, high-fiber foods, individuals can enjoy the benefits of better digestion, enhanced satiety, improved blood sugar control, and reduced risks of various health conditions.

History and Evolution of Dietary Fiber

The understanding and recognition of dietary fiber have undergone significant changes over centuries, transitioning from a neglected component to an essential part of a balanced diet.

Early Views and Neglect

In the early stages of nutrition science during the 19th century, dietary fiber was largely overlooked. Pioneering scientists such as William Prout and Justus von Liebig focused on proteins, fats, and carbohydrates as the primary nutrients essential for human health. Fiber, often termed as roughage, was considered non-essential and merely the indigestible part of plant foods.

Mid-20th Century Shifts

The mid-20th century saw a gradual shift in perspective. In the 1950s and 1960s, researchers began to notice the stark differences in disease prevalence between Western populations and those in parts of Africa and Asia, where diets were higher in unprocessed plant foods and thus fiber. However, it was the work of Dr. Denis Burkitt in the 1970s that truly revolutionized the understanding of dietary fiber. Burkitt observed that populations consuming high-fiber diets had lower incidences of conditions such as colon cancer, appendicitis, and heart disease. His research led to the formulation of the "fiber hypothesis," proposing that fiber played a crucial role in preventing these diseases.

Scientific Recognition and Public Awareness

Following Burkitt's influential studies, the scientific community began to conduct extensive research on dietary fiber. Studies started to differentiate between soluble and insoluble fibers, each with distinct health benefits. Soluble fiber was found to help lower cholesterol levels and regulate blood sugar, while insoluble fiber was linked to improved bowel health and prevention of constipation.

Public awareness of fiber's health benefits grew in the 1980s and 1990s, leading to dietary guidelines recommending increased fiber intake. Governments and health organizations worldwide began advocating for higher consumption of fruits, vegetables, whole grains, and legumes.

Modern Understanding and Current Trends

Today, dietary fiber is recognized as a vital nutrient with diverse health benefits. Modern research continues to uncover the complexities of fiber, including its role in gut health and its prebiotic properties, which support beneficial gut bacteria. The ongoing study of the gut microbiome has further highlighted fiber's importance in maintaining overall health.

Current dietary guidelines typically recommend a daily fiber intake of 25-30 grams, emphasizing the need for both soluble and insoluble fiber. The food industry has responded by fortifying products with fiber and marketing high-fiber foods as part of a healthy diet.

Importance of Fiber in the Diet

Fiber plays a critical role in maintaining overall health and well-being due to its multifaceted effects on various bodily functions. Here are several key reasons why fiber is important in the diet:

1. Digestive Health: Fiber is indispensable for proper digestive function. It adds bulk to stool, which aids in regular bowel movements and prevents constipation. By promoting the movement of waste through the digestive tract, fiber helps prevent gastrointestinal issues like diverticulosis and hemorrhoids. Adequate fiber intake ensures that the digestive system operates smoothly and efficiently.

2. Weight Management: Fiber-rich foods are typically low in calories but high in volume, making them ideal for weight management. These foods tend to be more filling, leading to a decreased appetite and reduced calorie intake overall. Additionally, fiber slows down the digestion process, prolonging the feeling of fullness after meals and preventing excessive snacking between meals. By helping to control appetite and regulate food intake, fiber contributes to maintaining a healthy body weight.

3. Blood Sugar Control: Fiber, especially soluble fiber found in foods like oats, beans, and fruits, plays a crucial role in regulating blood sugar levels. Soluble fiber forms a gel-like substance in the digestive tract, which slows down the absorption of glucose into the bloodstream. This gradual release of sugar helps prevent spikes in blood glucose

levels, making fiber-rich foods particularly beneficial for individuals with diabetes or those at risk of developing it. By promoting stable blood sugar levels, fiber reduces the risk of insulin resistance and related metabolic disorders.

4. Heart Health: Fiber is closely associated with cardiovascular health, primarily due to its ability to lower LDL cholesterol levels, often referred to as "bad" cholesterol. Soluble fiber binds to cholesterol particles in the digestive tract, preventing them from being absorbed into the bloodstream and ultimately facilitating their elimination from the body. By reducing LDL cholesterol levels, fiber helps prevent the buildup of plaque in the arteries, lowering the risk of heart disease and stroke. Furthermore, fiber-rich diets have been linked to lower blood pressure levels, further promoting cardiovascular well-being.

5. Gut Microbiome Support: Fiber serves as a prebiotic, nourishing the beneficial bacteria in the gut. These bacteria, collectively known as the gut microbiome, play a crucial role in various aspects of health, including digestion, immune function, and mental well-being. By providing substrate for the growth of beneficial bacteria, fiber helps maintain a diverse and balanced gut microbiome. A healthy gut microbiome is associated with reduced inflammation, improved nutrient absorption, enhanced immune response, and even better mental health outcomes.

SECTION 2: Types of Dietary Fiber: Soluble and Insoluble

Dietary fiber, the indigestible part of plant foods, can be broadly categorized into two main types: soluble fiber and insoluble fiber.

1. Soluble fiber:

- Soluble fiber dissolves in water to form a gel-like substance in the digestive tract. This gel helps to slow down the digestion process, leading to a more gradual release of nutrients into the bloodstream.

- One of the key benefits of soluble fiber is its ability to regulate blood sugar levels by slowing the absorption of sugar and improving insulin sensitivity.

- Soluble fiber also plays a role in lowering cholesterol levels by binding to cholesterol particles and promoting their excretion from the body, thus reducing the risk of heart disease.

- Good sources of soluble fiber include oats, barley, legumes (such as beans and lentils), fruits (such as apples, oranges, and berries), and some vegetables (like carrots and Brussels sprouts).

2. Insoluble fiber:

- Unlike soluble fiber, insoluble fiber does not dissolve in water and remains intact as it passes through the digestive system. Instead, it adds bulk to the stool, which helps to promote regular bowel movements and prevent constipation.

- Insoluble fiber also acts as a prebiotic, providing fuel for beneficial gut bacteria and supporting overall gut health.

- While insoluble fiber does not directly affect blood sugar or cholesterol levels, its role in promoting digestive regularity is essential for overall health.

- Common sources of insoluble fiber include whole grains (such as wheat bran, brown rice, and whole wheat bread), nuts, seeds, and many vegetables (including broccoli, cauliflower, and dark leafy greens).

Both types of fiber are important for maintaining a healthy digestive system and overall well-being. A balanced diet that includes a variety of fiber-rich foods ensures that you receive the benefits of both soluble and insoluble fiber.

Sources of Dietary Fiber

1. Fruits

- Apples: High in pectin, a type of soluble fiber, particularly beneficial for digestive health.

- Berries: Includes strawberries, raspberries, and blackberries, which are rich in both soluble and insoluble fiber.

- Oranges: Contain pectin and cellulose, providing a good mix of both types of fiber.

- Bananas: A good source of resistant starch and pectin, especially beneficial for gut health.

- Pears: High in pectin and a great source of both soluble and insoluble fiber.

2. Vegetables

- Broccoli: Contains a significant amount of fiber, including insoluble cellulose and soluble pectins.

- Carrots: Rich in cellulose, hemicellulose, and pectin, offering a good fiber blend.

- Brussels Sprouts: Packed with fiber, especially beneficial for maintaining a healthy digestive system.

- Spinach: Provides a good mix of soluble and insoluble fiber, aiding digestion.

- Sweet Potatoes: High in cellulose and pectin, making them a versatile fiber source.

3.Whole Grains

- Oats: Contain beta-glucan, a type of soluble fiber that helps reduce cholesterol levels.

- Brown Rice: Offers insoluble fiber, particularly beneficial for bowel health.

- Barley: Rich in beta-glucan, beneficial for blood sugar control and cholesterol management.

- Quinoa: A complete protein and high in both soluble and insoluble fiber.

- Whole Wheat Bread: Provides insoluble fiber from the bran, aiding digestion and preventing constipation.

4. Legumes

- Lentils: High in both soluble and insoluble fiber, making them excellent for digestive health and blood sugar control.

- Black Beans: Contain a good mix of fiber types, beneficial for heart health and digestion.

- Chickpeas: Rich in soluble fiber, particularly beneficial for lowering cholesterol.

- Kidney Beans: High in both types of fiber, promoting overall digestive health.

- Peas: Offer a mix of soluble and insoluble fiber, aiding in blood sugar regulation and digestive health.

5. Nuts and Seeds

- Almonds: High in both fiber and healthy fats, beneficial for heart health and digestion.

- Chia Seeds: Extremely rich in fiber, particularly soluble fiber, which helps with satiety and digestive health.

- Flaxseeds: High in soluble fiber, particularly beneficial for digestive and heart health.

- Sunflower Seeds: Provide a good amount of fiber along with healthy fats.

- Walnuts: Rich in fiber and omega-3 fatty acids, beneficial for heart and brain health.

6. Other Sources

- Popcorn: A whole grain and a great source of insoluble fiber when air-popped.

- Bran Cereal: Extremely high in fiber, especially beneficial for promoting regular bowel movements.

- Psyllium Husk: A highly concentrated source of soluble fiber, often used as a dietary supplement.

- Avocado: Rich in both soluble and insoluble fiber, also provides healthy fats.

- Edamame: High in fiber and protein, beneficial for digestive health and weight management.

These sources offer a variety of fiber types and benefits, making it easier to incorporate sufficient fiber into the diet through diverse and nutritious foods.

How Fiber Affects the Body

Dietary fiber affects the body in several important ways:

1. Digestive Health: Fiber adds bulk to the stool, which helps regulate bowel movements and prevents constipation. It also aids in preventing conditions like diverticulosis and hemorrhoids.

2. Blood Sugar Control: Soluble fiber slows the digestion and absorption of carbohydrates, which helps prevent spikes in blood sugar levels and improves overall glycemic control. This is particularly beneficial for individuals with diabetes.

3. Cholesterol Management: Soluble fiber binds to bile acids in the intestine, which are then excreted. This process forces the liver to use cholesterol to produce more bile acids, thus lowering levels of LDL (bad) cholesterol and reducing the risk of cardiovascular diseases.

4. Weight Management: High-fiber foods are generally more filling than low-fiber foods, which can help control appetite and reduce overall calorie intake. Fiber slows digestion, prolonging the feeling of fullness and reducing the likelihood of overeating.

5. Gut Health: Fiber acts as a prebiotic, supporting the growth of beneficial bacteria in the gut. A healthy gut microbiome is essential for a strong immune system, effective digestion, and overall health. It can also help reduce the risk of inflammatory bowel disease (IBD) and irritable bowel syndrome (IBS).

6. Cancer Prevention: Some studies suggest that a high-fiber diet may help reduce the risk of certain types of cancer, particularly colorectal cancer, by promoting regular bowel movements and reducing the time harmful substances spend in the intestine.

7. Detoxification: Fiber helps the body eliminate waste products more efficiently, which can reduce the burden on the liver and kidneys and promote overall detoxification.

SECTION 3: Health Benefits of a High-Fiber Diet

1. Digestive Health

- Promotes regular bowel movements: Fiber adds bulk to the stool and helps it pass more easily through the digestive tract, preventing constipation.

- Prevents constipation and hemorrhoids: By softening the stool and making it easier to pass, fiber reduces the strain on the digestive system, which can help prevent hemorrhoids and other related issues.

- Reduces the risk of diverticulitis: High-fiber diets can help prevent the formation of small pouches in the colon (diverticula) and reduce inflammation of these pouches.

2. Weight Management

- Enhances feelings of fullness: Fiber-rich foods tend to be more filling than low-fiber foods, helping you feel satisfied for longer periods and reducing the likelihood of overeating.

- Reduces overall calorie intake: High-fiber foods are often less energy-dense, meaning they provide fewer calories for the same volume of food, which can aid in weight loss and management.

3. Cardiovascular Benefits

- Lowers cholesterol levels: Soluble fiber can help lower total blood cholesterol levels by binding to cholesterol particles in the digestive system and removing them from the body.

- Reduces the risk of heart disease: By lowering bad cholesterol (LDL) and improving overall heart health, fiber contributes to a reduced risk of developing heart disease.

4. Blood Sugar Control

- Stabilizes blood sugar levels: Soluble fiber slows the absorption of sugar, which can help improve blood sugar levels and prevent spikes.

- Lowers the risk of type 2 diabetes: Regular consumption of high-fiber foods can help maintain healthy blood glucose levels and reduce the risk of developing type 2 diabetes.

5. Other Health Benefits

- Reduces the risk of certain cancers: High fiber intake has been associated with a lower risk of colorectal cancer, possibly due to its ability to accelerate the removal of waste from the intestines.

- Supports a healthy gut microbiome: Fiber serves as a prebiotic, providing food for beneficial gut bacteria, which in turn support overall digestive health and boost the immune system.

- May reduce inflammation: Diets rich in fiber have been linked to lower levels of inflammation in the body, which is beneficial for preventing chronic diseases such as arthritis and other inflammatory conditions.

By incorporating more fiber into your diet, you can reap these numerous health benefits, contributing to overall well-being and long-term health.

Practical Tips for Incorporating Fiber into Your Diet

1. Start Your Day with Fiber

- High-Fiber Breakfasts: Begin your day with a fiber-rich breakfast like oatmeal topped with fruits, whole-grain cereals, or smoothies with added chia seeds or flaxseeds. These options can help keep you full until your next meal.

2. Choose Whole Grains

- Switch to Whole Grains: Replace refined grains with whole grains such as brown rice, quinoa, whole wheat bread, and whole grain pasta. These options are higher in fiber and more nutritious overall.

3. Eat More Fruits and Vegetables

- Five-a-Day: Aim to fill half your plate with fruits and vegetables. Incorporate a variety of colors and types to ensure you get a range of nutrients and fibers.

4. Snack Smart

- Fiber-Rich Snacks: Choose high-fiber snacks like raw vegetables with hummus, fresh fruits, nuts, and seeds. These snacks can help maintain energy levels and reduce the temptation to indulge in less healthy options.

5. Include Legumes in Your Diet

- Beans and Lentils: Add beans, lentils, and other legumes to soups, stews, salads, and casseroles. They are excellent sources of both fiber and protein, making meals more satisfying.

6. Hydrate Well

- Drink Plenty of Water: Fiber works best when it absorbs water. Drinking enough fluids is essential to prevent digestive discomfort and support the effective movement of fiber through your digestive system.

7. Read Nutrition Labels

- Check for Fiber Content: When shopping, read nutrition labels to choose products with higher fiber content. Look for breads, cereals, and snacks that offer at least 3 grams of fiber per serving.

8. Gradually Increase Fiber Intake

- Avoid Sudden Changes: To prevent bloating and gas, increase your fiber intake gradually over a few weeks. This allows your digestive system to adjust to the higher fiber levels.

Fiber for Different Life Stages

Dietary needs change throughout life, and fiber is no exception. Here's how to tailor fiber intake for different life stages to ensure optimal health and well-being.

Children and Teens

Nutritional Needs:

Children and teens require adequate fiber to support growth and development. Fiber aids in maintaining healthy digestion, preventing constipation, and fostering a balanced gut microbiome.

Recommended Intake:

- Children (1-3 years): 19 grams/day

- Children (4-8 years): 25 grams/day

- Boys (9-13 years): 31 grams/day

- Girls (9-13 years): 26 grams/day

- Boys (14-18 years): 38 grams/day

- Girls (14-18 years): 26 grams/day

Tips for Incorporation:

- Introduce a variety of fruits, vegetables, whole grains, and legumes.

- Encourage whole fruit over fruit juices to increase fiber intake.

- Include high-fiber snacks such as air-popped popcorn, nuts, and whole grain crackers.

Adults

Nutritional Needs:

Fiber continues to play a crucial role in maintaining digestive health, managing weight, and reducing the risk of chronic diseases such as heart disease, type 2 diabetes, and certain cancers.

Recommended Intake:

- Men (19-50 years): 38 grams/day

- Women (19-50 years): 25 grams/day

- Men (51+ years): 30 grams/day

- Women (51+ years): 21 grams/day

Tips for Incorporation:

- Start the day with a high-fiber breakfast like oatmeal topped with berries and nuts.

- Choose whole grain products over refined grains.

- Add beans and lentils to soups, salads, and stews.

Seniors

Nutritional Needs:

As people age, digestive health can become more delicate, and the risk of constipation increases. Fiber helps maintain regularity and supports overall health.

Recommended Intake:

- Men (51+ years): 30 grams/day

- Women (51+ years): 21 grams/day

Tips for Incorporation:

- Opt for cooked vegetables, which are easier to digest, alongside raw options.

- Include a variety of fiber-rich foods to ensure adequate nutrient intake.

- Stay hydrated, as fiber works best with sufficient fluid intake.

Pregnant and Nursing Women

Nutritional Needs:

Fiber is essential during pregnancy and lactation to prevent constipation, manage healthy weight gain, and ensure a diverse and healthy gut microbiome, which is beneficial for both mother and baby.

Recommended Intake:

- Pregnant women: 28 grams/day

- Nursing women: 29 grams/day

Tips for Incorporation:

- Consume a balanced diet rich in whole grains, fruits, vegetables, and legumes.

- Monitor fiber intake to avoid excessive gas and bloating.

- Gradually increase fiber intake to allow the digestive system to adjust.

General Tips for All Life Stages

1. Variety is Key:

   - Incorporate a range of fiber sources to benefit from different types of fiber and nutrients.

2. Hydration:

   - Drink plenty of water throughout the day to help fiber move through the digestive system smoothly.

3. Gradual Increase:

   - Increase fiber intake gradually to prevent digestive discomfort.

4. Balanced Diet:

- Ensure a balanced diet that includes all essential nutrients alongside fiber for overall health.

By tailoring fiber intake to the specific needs of different life stages, individuals can optimize their health and well-being throughout their lives.

SECTION 4: Weight Management on the Fiber Diet

anaging weight effectively is a common goal for many individuals, and incorporating dietary fiber into your routine can be a powerful tool in achieving and maintaining a healthy weight. The Fiber Diet emphasizes the consumption of high-fiber foods, which not only offer numerous health benefits but also play a crucial role in weight management. Here's how fiber helps with weight control and some practical tips to incorporate more fiber into your diet.

How Fiber Aids in Weight Management

1. Increased Satiety

- Feeling Full Longer: Fiber-rich foods tend to be more filling than low-fiber foods. Soluble fiber absorbs water and forms a gel-like substance in the gut, slowing down digestion and promoting a sense of fullness. This can help reduce overall calorie intake by curbing hunger between meals.

- Slower Eating: High-fiber foods often require more chewing, which can slow down eating and give your body more time to register fullness, potentially leading to reduced food intake.

2. Lower Energy Density

- Fewer Calories per Bite: Foods high in fiber typically have lower energy density, meaning they provide fewer calories per gram compared to low-fiber foods. This allows you to eat satisfying portions without consuming excessive calories.

3. Improved Blood Sugar Control

- Stable Blood Sugar Levels: Soluble fiber slows the absorption of sugar, helping to maintain stable blood glucose levels. This can prevent spikes and crashes that often lead to cravings and overeating.

4. Enhanced Gut Health

- Healthy Gut Microbiome: Fiber acts as a prebiotic, feeding the beneficial bacteria in your gut. A healthy gut microbiome is associated with better digestion, improved metabolism, and a lower risk of obesity.

Sample Fiber-Rich Meal Plan for Weight Management

Breakfast:

- Oatmeal topped with berries and a tablespoon of chia seeds

- A glass of water

Mid-Morning Snack:

- An apple with a handful of almonds

Lunch:

- Quinoa salad with mixed vegetables, chickpeas, and a light vinaigrette

- A glass of water

Afternoon Snack:

- Carrot sticks with hummus

Dinner:

- Grilled chicken breast with steamed broccoli and a side of brown rice

- A glass of water

Evening Snack:

- A small bowl of mixed berries

By following these guidelines and incorporating fiber-rich foods into your diet, you can effectively manage your weight while enjoying a variety of delicious and nutritious meals. Remember, consistency is key, and making small, sustainable changes to your eating habits can lead to long-term success.

SECTION 5: Getting Started with the Fiber Diet

Embarking on a fiber-rich diet is a transformative journey towards better health and well-being. Whether you're aiming to improve your digestive health, manage weight, or prevent chronic diseases, increasing your fiber intake is a key step. This chapter will guide you through the initial stages of adopting a fiber diet, helping you to assess your current intake, set realistic goals, and debunk common myths.

Assessing Your Current Fiber Intake

Before making any dietary changes, it's essential to understand your starting point. Here's how you can assess your current fiber intake:

1. Keep a Food Diary: Record everything you eat and drink for a week. Include portion sizes and specific details about your meals and snacks.

2. Analyze Fiber Content: Use nutrition labels or an online food database to determine the fiber content of each item. Pay special attention to fruits, vegetables, whole grains, legumes, nuts, and seeds.

3. Calculate Your Daily Intake: Sum up the fiber content from your food diary to get an estimate of your daily fiber intake.

Setting Realistic Goals

Once you have a clear picture of your current fiber intake, you can set achievable goals. Here are some tips for setting realistic and sustainable fiber goals:

1. Know the Recommended Intake: The recommended daily intake of fiber is about 25 grams for women and 38 grams for men. However, individual needs may vary based on age, sex, and health status.

2. Start Slow: If your current intake is significantly lower than the recommended amount, increase your fiber gradually. Adding too much fiber too quickly can lead to digestive discomfort.

3. Set Incremental Goals: Aim to increase your fiber intake by 3-5 grams per week until you reach

your target. This gradual approach allows your
digestive system to adjust.

SECTION 6: Common Myths and Misconceptions

There are many myths about fiber that can create confusion. Let's debunk some of the most common misconceptions:

1. Myth: All Fiber is the Same

- Fact: There are two main types of fiber—soluble and insoluble. Both types have different benefits and sources. Soluble fiber dissolves in water and helps lower cholesterol and blood sugar levels, while insoluble fiber adds bulk to the stool and aids in regular bowel movements.

2. Myth: Fiber Supplements are Just as Good as Food Sources

- Fact: While fiber supplements can be helpful, they should not replace food sources. Whole foods provide additional nutrients and health benefits that supplements alone cannot offer.

3. Myth: High-Fiber Diets are Boring and Tasteless

- Fact: A high-fiber diet can be delicious and varied. There are countless ways to incorporate fiber-rich foods into your meals, from fresh fruits and vegetables to whole grains and legumes.

Practical Tips for Increasing Fiber Intake

Here are some practical tips to help you incorporate more fiber into your diet:

1. Start Your Day with Fiber: Choose a high-fiber breakfast such as oatmeal topped with berries, whole grain cereal, or a smoothie with added flaxseeds or chia seeds.

2. Snack Smart: Opt for fiber-rich snacks like fresh fruits, raw vegetables with hummus, popcorn, or a handful of nuts and seeds.

3. Incorporate Legumes: Add beans, lentils, and peas to soups, salads, and main dishes. They are excellent sources of both soluble and insoluble fiber.

4. Choose Whole Grains: Replace refined grains with whole grains such as brown rice, quinoa, barley, and whole wheat products.

5. Boost Fiber in Baked Goods: Use whole grain flour and add ingredients like oats, bran, and seeds to your baking recipes.

Staying Motivated

Staying motivated is crucial for long-term success. Here are some strategies to keep you on track:

1. Track Your Progress: Continue keeping a food diary and monitor your fiber intake. Celebrate your achievements and adjust your goals as needed.

2. Join a Support Group: Find a community of like-minded individuals who are also focusing on a high-fiber diet. Share tips, recipes, and experiences.

3. Experiment with Recipes: Keep your meals exciting by trying new recipes and exploring different cuisines that emphasize fiber-rich ingredients.

By assessing your current fiber intake, setting realistic goals, and gradually increasing your consumption, you can successfully transition to a fiber-rich diet. Remember, the journey to better health is a marathon, not a sprint. With patience and persistence, you'll reap the numerous benefits that dietary fiber has to offer.

SECTION 7: WHOLESOME RECIPES FOR HIGH FIBER DIET

WHOLESOME RECIPES FOR BREAKFAST

Veggie Pocket

Things Needed

for 1 serving

2 teaspoons olive oil

½ red bell pepper, sliced

¼ cup canned black bean(40 g), drained and rinsed

¼ cup frozen corn(45 g), thawed

½ small yellow onion, thinly sliced

2 eggs

¼ teaspoon salt

¼ teaspoon ground black pepper

¼ cup shredded cheddar cheese(25 g)

1 whole wheat tortilla, medium

Method

Heat olive oil in a nonstick skillet over medium heat.

Add the bell pepper, black beans, corn, and onions, and cook until caramelized, about 5 minutes.

Remove the vegetables from the pan and set aside.

Reduce heat to low, and eggs, and sprinkle with salt and pepper. Cook, stirring constantly, until barely set, about 2 minutes.

Place the vegetables, scrambled eggs, and cheese in the center of a tortilla, and fold the sides into the center, completely covering the filling.

Add the quesadilla, seam side down, to the skillet and cook over medium heat until the outside is toasted and cheese is melted.

Enjoy!

Cinnamon Roll-Stuffed Baked Apples

Things Needed

for 5 servings

1 8-count can of cinnamon rolls, icing reserved

8 baking apples, such as Gala

melted butter, for brushing

brown sugar, for sprinkling

1 teaspoon ground cinnamon, for sprinkling

Method

Preheat the oven to 350°F (180°C).

Slice off the top of each apple and hollow out the inside using a melon baller, leaving a thicker base at the bottom and being careful not to cut through the sides.

Add a bit of melted butter and a sprinkle of brown sugar and cinnamon to the inside of each apple, then brush to coat evenly.

Place a cinnamon roll in each apple. Place the apples in a baking dish so they remain upright.

Bake the apples for15 minutes, then cover loosely with foil and bake for another 25-30 minutes, until the cinnamon rolls are baked through.

Remove from the oven and drizzle with the reserved icing. Serve warm.

Enjoy!

Pesto & Parmesan Avocado Toast

Things Needed

for 1 serving

bread, toasted

½ avocado, sliced

2 tablespoons pesto

2 tablespoons parmesan cheese, shaved

Method

Spread pesto on toast.

Top with sliced avocado and shaved parmesan cheese.

Enjoy!

Eggs Benedict With Spinach

Things Needed

for 2 servings

FLORENTINE BENEDICT

1 english muffin

1 tablespoon butter

2 eggs

1 tablespoon olive oil

1 cup fresh spinach(40 g)

2 pieces canadian bacon

chive

HOLLANDAISE

2 egg yolks

1 tablespoon lemon juice

1 teaspoon salt

1 pinch cayenne

½ cup butter(115 g), melted

Method

Preheat oven to 400°F (200°C).

In a sauté pan, heat the olive oil and add the spinach and a pinch of salt. Sauté until wilted. Set aside.

Butter the English muffin and toast in the oven for 5-10 minutes or until brown.

Heat a pot of water over medium heat. With a wooden spoon, swirl the water in the same direction.

Quickly add the egg into the center of the swirling water, cover, and cook for 3-5 minutes or until egg white is set and yolk is still runny.

Remove egg from water with a slotted spoon and set aside.

In a blender, add the egg yolks and pulse for one minute. Add in the lemon juice, salt, and cayenne and run the blender. Slowly add in the melted butter and continue to blend until the mixture lightens in color. Add more melted butter for thinner consistency.

Assemble the Benedict by layering the english muffin with the bacon, spinach, poached egg, and hollandaise sauce.

Top with fresh chives.

Enjoy!

Banana Matcha Smoothie

Things Needed

for 2 servings

1 banana, sliced

1 tablespoon matcha powder, plus more for serving

1 cup almond milk(240 mL)

1 cup fresh spinach(40 g)

2 cups ice(480 g)

Method

Add the banana, matcha, almond milk, spinach, and ice to a blender.

Blend until smooth.

Serve in a glass topped with a sprinkle of matcha.

Enjoy!

Crispy Cheesy Hash Brown Egg Bake

Things Needed

for 6 servings

4 lb russet potato(1.8 kg)

salt, to taste

pepper, to taste

1 tablespoon garlic powder

¼ teaspoon cayenne pepper

1 teaspoon onion powder

1 cup shredded parmesan cheese(100 g)

¼ cup olive oil(60 mL)

12 slices cheddar cheese, cut into 1x3in (2x7 cm) strips

12 slices deli ham, cut into 1x3in (2x7 cm) strips

6 large eggs

fresh chive, chopped, for garnish

Method

Preheat the oven to 400°F (200°C). Grease a 9x13-inch (23x33-cm) baking dish with non-stick cooking spray

Peel the potatoes, then shred on the large holes of a box grater. Transfer to a large bowl of water and swirl around to remove excess starch. Drain and rinse, then place the potatoes in a clean kitchen towel and squeeze until they're completely dry.

Add the shredded potatoes to a clean, large bowl with the salt, pepper, garlic powder, cayenne, onion powder, Parmesan cheese, and olive oil. Toss until fully combined.

Transfer the potato mixture to the baking dish. Spread evenly.

Bake for 1½ hours, or until the potatoes are tender throughout and golden brown on the top and bottom.

Press the bottom of a glass into the potato mixture to create 6 evenly spaced wells.

Shingle slices of cheddar cheese and ham around the wells, then crack an egg into each one.

Bake for 15 minutes more, or until the cheese melts and the egg whites are set. The egg yolks should still be slightly soft.

Serve and sprinkle with chives, if desired.

Enjoy!

Sweet Potato Black Bean Hash

Things Needed

for 4 servings

4 tablespoons olive oil

3 cups sweet potato(600 g), diced, about 2 large potatoes

½ yellow onion, diced

1 red bell pepper, sliced

salt, to taste

pepper, to taste

½ tablespoon paprika

1 teaspoon cumin

2 cups spinach(80 g)

15 oz black beans(425 g), 1 can

Method

Heat olive oil on medium heat in a 4-quart chicken fryer. Add sweet potatoes, onion, pepper, salt, pepper, paprika, and cumin, and stir. Cook for 10 minutes, occasionally stirring.

Add spinach and cook for an additional five minutes.

Lastly, add the black beans and stir until all **Things Needed** are well-blended.

Serve with toppings of your choice. We topped our hash with an egg and avocado slices.

Enjoy!

Avocado Egg Cups

Things Needed

for 4 servings

2 ripe avocados

4 large eggs

OPTIONAL TOPPINGS

tomato, diced

fresh basil, chopped

feta cheese, crumbled

bell pepper, diced

onion, diced

turkey bacon, chopped

chive, chopped

salt, to taste

pepper, to taste

Method

Preheat the oven to 425°F (220°C).

Cut the avocados in half and carefully remove the pits.

Scoop out 1-2 tablespoons of avocado from the center of each half (save it for another meal!).

Transfer the avocado halves to a baking sheet and carefully crack an egg into each avocado cup. If the divot is too small, it may be easier to separate the egg yolks and whites before placing them in the avocado.

Add your favorite topping combo, such as tomato and basil, feta cheese, bell pepper and onion, and bacon and chives. Season with salt and pepper to taste

Bake for 18 minutes, or until the egg whites have cooked completely.

Enjoy!

Homemade Muesli

Things Needed

for 6 cups

4 cups rolled oats(320 g)

1 cup raisin(150 g)

1 cup peanuts(125 g), chopped

½ cup sunflower seeds(70 g)

2 tablespoons chia seeds, optional

1 teaspoon cinnamon, optional

Method

Combine the rolled oats, raisins, peanuts, sunflower seeds, chia seeds, and cinnamon in a large bowl until evenly mixed.

Store in airtight container for up to 6 months.

Serve as desired.

Enjoy!

Potato Flower Breakfast Cups

Things Needed

for 12 potato cups

5 medium russet potatoes

2 teaspoons salt, divided, plus more to taste

1 teaspoon pepper

1 teaspoon paprika

1 teaspoon garlic powder

1 teaspoon fresh parsley

1 tablespoon vegetable oil

2 cups shredded cheese blend(200 g)

5 strips bacon, cooked and finely chopped

12 large eggs

Method

Preheat the oven to 400°F (200°C).

With a mandolin or a sharp knife, carefully cut the potatoes into $\frac{1}{16}$-inch (1 mm) thick slices.

Add the potato slices to a large bowl and cover with water. Toss the potatoes around to remove excess starch, then drain.

Add 1 teaspoon of salt, the pepper, paprika, and garlic powder and toss the potatoes until evenly coated.

Add the oil to a small bowl. Dip a paper towel in the oil and grease the cups of a 12-cup muffin tin.

Arrange 5 potatoes around the sides of a muffin cup, overlapping slightly. Place 1 slice on the bottom to create a flower. Repeat with the remaining potato slices. Sprinkle shredded cheese over the potato cups.

Bake for 10 minutes.

Remove the potato cups from the oven and reduce the oven temperature to 300°F (150°C).

Sprinkle bacon over the cheese. Add an egg to each cup. Sprinkle with salt.

Bake for another 20-25 minutes, or until the egg whites are mostly cooked.

Serve warm.

Enjoy!

Tropical Fruit Salad

Things Needed

for 4 servings

2 oranges, peeled and halved

12 oz fresh strawberry (340 g), quartered

2 mangoes, chopped

4 kiwis, peeled and chopped, or sliced

DRESSING

3 tablespoons lime juice

1 tablespoon maple syrup

Method

Combine all the **Things Needed** above in a large bowl.

Mix the dressing **Things Needed** together and spread over fruit, mix well.

Enjoy!

Cheddar-Stuffed Biscuits

Things Needed

for 8 biscuits

BISCUITS

2 cups bisquick(240 g)

4 tablespoons butter

⅔ cup milk(160 mL)

1 teaspoon dried parsley

1 cup shredded cheddar cheese(100 g)

8 cubes cheddar cheese

BUTTER TOPPING

2 tablespoons butter, melted

½ teaspoon garlic powder

½ teaspoon old bay seasoning

Method

Preheat the oven to 450°F (230°C).

In a large bowl, combine the Bisquick and butter until crumbly.

Add the milk, dried parsley and shredded cheddar and mix to combine. The dough will be sticky.

Take a handful of dough, flatten, and place a cube of cheese in the middle. Roll the dough around the cube of cheese. Place on a parchment-lined baking sheet and repeat with the remaining dough and cheese.

Bake for 10-15 minutes, until golden brown.

While the biscuits are baking, make the butter topping. Combine the melted butter, garlic powder, and Old Bay seasoning.

Once the biscuits are done baking, brush the butter topping over each biscuit.

Enjoy!

WHOLESOME RECIPES FOR LUNCH

Crunchy Thai Salad

Things Needed

for 1 serving

DRESSING

1 tablespoon peanut butter

1 tablespoon soy sauce

½ teaspoon sriracha

SALAD

½ cup cabbage(50 g), chopped

½ cup broccoli floret(75 g), broken up

½ red bell pepper, chopped

½ cup fresh chives(20 g), chopped

½ cup carrot(55 g), shredded

¼ cup peanuts(30 g), chopped

1 cup lettuce(75 g)

Method

In a large mason jar, add the peanut butter, soy sauce and sriracha and stir to combine.

Add the cabbage, broccoli florets, bell pepper, chives, carrots, peanuts, and lettuce and screw on the lid.

Store in the refrigerator until ready to eat, up to 5 days.

Give the mason jar a good shake to mix and use a fork or spoon to stir as needed.

Enjoy!

Stuffed Shells

Things Needed

for 8 servings

1 teaspoon kosher salt, plus more for boiling

1 package jumbo shell

1 tablespoon olive oil, plus more for greasing

3 cloves garlic, minced

4 cups fresh spinach(160 g), packed

1 container ricotta cheese

10 large eggs

1 cup finely grated parmesan cheese(125 g)

1 teaspoon freshly ground black pepper

½ teaspoon red pepper flakes

3 cups marinara sauce(720 g), divided

1 cup shredded mozzarella cheese(100 g)

fresh basil leaf, for garnish

Method

Preheat the oven to 375°F (190°C).

Bring a large pot of salted water to a boil over high heat. Add the jumbo shells and cook according to the package instructions until al dente. Drain the jumbo shells through a colander.

Heat the olive oil in a large pan over medium-high heat. Once the oil begins to shimmer, add the garlic and stir until aromatic, about 30 seconds. Add the spinach and cook until just wilted down, about 1 minute. Remove the pan from the heat and let the spinach cool to room temperature, then roughly chop on a cutting board.

In a medium bowl, mix together the ricotta and egg. Add the chopped spinach, Parmesan, 1 teaspoon kosher salt, the black pepper, and red pepper flakes and stir to combine.

Fill the jumbo shells with the ricotta mixture.

Grease a 9 x 13-inch baking dish with olive oil. Spread 2 cups of marinara on the bottom of the pan.

Arrange the stuffed shells in a single layer over the marinara sauce. Spread the remaining 1 cup of marinara over the shells and top with the mozzarella.

Cover the baking dish with foil and bake for 20 minutes. Uncover the pan and continue baking until the cheese has melted and is golden brown, about 15 minutes.

Garnish with the basil and serve immediately.

Enjoy!

Thai Quinoa Salad

Things Needed

for 2 servings

SALAD

1 cup water(235 mL)

1 cup vegetable stock(235 mL)

1 cup quinoa(170 g)

2 carrots, shredded

1 red bell pepper, diced

1 cucumber, quartered

1 cup red cabbage(100 g), shredded

½ small red onion, diced

½ cup edamame(75 g)

green onion, to serve

½ cup crushed peanut(60 g), to serve

DRESSING

½ cup water(120 mL)

1 teaspoon sesame oil

1 tablespoon soy sauce

1 tablespoon ginger, grated

2 teaspoons olive oil

1 tablespoon honey

¼ cup peanut butter(60 g)

Method

In a small saucepan, bring water and vegetable stock to a boil, then add quinoa. Cover and simmer for 12-15 minutes.

In a bowl, combine quinoa, carrots, red pepper, cucumber, purple cabbage, and edamame.

In a small bowl, mix water, sesame oil, soy sauce, ginger, olive oil, honey, and peanut butter. Drizzle dressing over the quinoa.

Top with green onions and crushed peanuts.

Enjoy!

Chicken Fajita Soup

Things Needed

for 6 servings

2 lb chicken(1 kg), cut of your choice, diced

2 teaspoons chili powder

2 teaspoons cumin

½ teaspoon pepper

3 cloves garlic cloves, minced

1 onion, chopped

3 bell peppers, chopped

2 limes

14 oz crushed tomato(395 g)

48 fl oz chicken broth(1 ½ L)

½ cup cream(120 mL)

6 corn soft tortillas

1 cup frozen corn(175 g)

Method

In a 5-quart Dutch oven coated with oil, cook chicken, chili powder, cumin, and pepper for 3 minutes.

Add the garlic, onion, and bell peppers, and cook until the onions are clear.

Add the juice of 2 limes, crushed tomato, chicken broth, and cream, and bring to a boil.

Submerge the corn and corn tortillas in the soup.

Reduce heat, cover, and simmer for 20 minutes.

Stir to break up the tortillas before serving. Top with avocado, cilantro, and cotija cheese if you want!

Enjoy!

Chicken Pot Pie

Things Needed

for 4 servings

4 tablespoons unsalted butter, at room temperature

4 tablespoons all-purpose flour, plus more for dusting

2 cups chicken broth(480 g), good-quality

salt, to taste

freshly ground black pepper, to taste

1 pinch cayenne pepper, optional, to taste

2 tablespoons heavy cream, plus more for egg wash

2 lb cooked boneless, skinless chicken(910 g), shredded

½ lb carrot(225 g), peeled, cut into 1/2-inch (1cm) pieces

½ lb red-skinned potato(225 g), cut into 1/2-inch (1cm) pieces

½ cup frozen peas(75 g), or shelled fresh peas

½ lb puff pastry(225 g), defrosted following package instructions

1 black truffle, optional, to taste

1 large egg

Method

Melt the butter in a large, deep saucepan.

Add the flour and whisk to ensure there are no lumps before adding the chicken stock. Cook for 5-10 minutes while continuously stirring.

Check the consistency by dipping the back of a spoon into the sauce and running your finger along the spoon. You want the sauce to cling to the spoon and not run over the swipe you made.

Continue to cook and stir the sauce over medium heat until you reach the correct consistency. Season with the salt, pepper, and cayenne (if using). Taste the sauce and see if your sauce needs more seasoning.

Add the cream and stir to combine.

Add the shredded chicken, carrots, potatoes, and peas to the sauce. Cook the vegetables in the sauce for 2-3 minutes.

Transfer the filling to a clean bowl and chill in the refrigerator for 1 hour, or until cool.

Preheat the oven to 400°F (200°C).

Roll out the puff pastry, using a bit of extra flour to ensure the pastry doesn't stick to your work surface. Use a bowl or plate about an inch (2 cm) larger than the dish you are cooking your pot pie in as a guide to cut out your pastry.

Carefully spoon the chilled filling into oven-proof serving bowls.

Break the egg in a small bowl and add a tablespoon of water or cream. Whisk with a fork.

Brush the egg wash on the edges and rim of your dishes.

If desired, shave truffles over the filling. Lay the pastry rounds over the top, being careful not to stretch the pastry. Seal the edges of the pastry by lightly pushing it onto the rim of your dish to make sure it is secure.

Brush the top and sides with more egg wash.

Place the pot pies on a large baking sheet and bake for 25-35 minutes, until the pastry is a nice golden, dark brown and there are no more grayish raw patches.

Let cool for 5 minutes before serving.

Enjoy!

Chicken Salad Sandwich

Things Needed

for 1 serving

½ cup shredded chicken(125 g)

2 tablespoons celery, diced

1 tablespoon white onion, finely diced

6 cherry tomatoes, sliced in half

2 tablespoons apple, diced

3 tablespoons greek yogurt

salt, to taste

pepper, to taste

2 pieces whole wheat bread

1 leaf romaine lettuce

Method

In a bowl, combine chicken, celery, onion, sliced tomatoes, apple, yogurt, salt and pepper.

Spread the chicken salad on one of the pieces of bread and place the lettuce on the other piece. Top with desired condiments and bring the two pieces of bread together. Cut in half and place in a reusable container with some fruits and veggies.

Enjoy!

Vegetarian Grain Bowl Meal Prep

Things Needed

for 4 servings

ROASTED CHICKPEA & VEGGIE BROWN RICE BOWL

1 sweet potato, peeled and chopped into bite-size pieces

½ lb brussels sprouts(230 g), trimmed and halved

1 yellow bell pepper, roughly chopped

½ red onion, roughly chopped

15 oz can of chickpeas, drained and rinsed

olive oil, to taste

salt, to taste

pepper, to taste

paprika, to taste

2 cups brown rice(460 g), cooked

ROASTED VEGGIE QUINOA BOWL

2 carrots, sliced

1 head broccoli, cut into florets

1 red bell pepper, roughly chopped

½ head red cabbage, sliced

1 cup sugar snap peas(65 g)

olive oil, to taste

salt, to taste

pepper, to taste

garlic powder, to taste

onion powder, to taste

2 cups quinoa(340 g), cooked

CILANTRO LIME DRESSING

¼ cup plain greek yogurt(75 g)

2 tablespoons lime juice

1 tablespoon fresh cilantro, chopped

salt, to taste

pepper, to taste

SOY MAPLE DRESSING

¼ cup soy sauce(60 mL)

2 tablespoons pure maple syrup

1 teaspoon fresh ginger, minced

1 teaspoon garlic, minced

pepper, to taste

Method

Preheat the oven to 425°F (220°C). Line 2 baking sheets with parchment paper.

On 1 baking sheet, season the vegetables and chickpeas for the Roasted Chickpea & Veggie

Brown Rice Bowl with olive oil, salt, pepper, and paprika.

On the other baking sheet, season the vegetables for the Roasted Veggie Quinoa Bowl with olive oil, salt, pepper, garlic powder, and onion powder.

Bake for 15 -20 minutes, or until the vegetables are roasted to your liking.

Fill 2 glass storage bowls with 1 cup cooked brown rice each. Fill 2 more glass storage bowls with 1 cup cooked quinoa each.

Fill the brown rice bowls with the roasted chickpea and vegetables. Fill the quinoa bowls with the other roasted vegetables.

Mix the cilantro-lime dressing **Things Needed** and split the dressing between 2 small glass containers. Store in the refrigerator with the roasted vegetable and chickpea bowls for up to 4 days.

Mix the soy-maple dressing **Things Needed** and split the dressing between 2 small glass containers. Store in the refrigerator with the roasted vegetable quinoa bowls for up to 4 days.

To serve, remove the containers with the dressing and heat the bowls in the microwave for 1 minute. Pour the dressing on top and mix everything together.

Enjoy!

Pesto Asparagus And Sun-Dried Tomato Pasta

Things Needed

for 4 servings

3 cloves garlic

15 spears asparagus

1 teaspoon olive oil

1 teaspoon salt, to taste

1 teaspoon pepper, to taste

8 oz penne pasta(225 g)

PESTO

4 cups fresh basil leaves(160 g)

⅓ cup pine nuts(40 g)

2 cloves garlic

½ cup olive oil(120 mL)

½ cup parmesan cheese(55 g)

1 teaspoon salt

½ cup sun-dried tomato(100 g)

½ cup parmesan cheese, optional

Method

Preheat oven to 425°F/220°C.

In a large pot, bring 4 quarts of water to a rolling boil.

Remove the woody ends of the asparagus and discard. Cut the remaining spears into quarters and place on a baking sheet. Drizzle olive oil, salt, and pepper over the asparagus and toss so each piece is evenly coated. Bake for 10 minutes.

In the boiling water, cook the penne for 10–12 minutes, or until al dente, and drain.

Using a blender or food processor, blend basil, pine nuts, garlic, and olive oil until it becomes a paste. Add in Parmesan and salt and blend.

In a large bowl, combine cooked pasta, sun-dried tomatoes, roasted asparagus, and pesto (about 3 hefty tablespoons). Toss together and serve hot or cold, and top with Parmesan cheese.

Enjoy!

Onigirazu (Rice Sandwich)

Things Needed

for 1 serving

1 sheet nori

1 cup rice(230 g), cooked

salt, to taste

2 teaspoons sesame seeds

2 tablespoons salmon, cooked

1 shiso leaf

Method

Set the nori sheet on a clean work surface. Season the rice with a pinch of salt.

Place half of the rice in the center of the nori and sprinkle with sesame seeds. Place the cooked salmon and shiso leaf on top.

Top with the remaining rice, then wrap the nori into a square and flip upside down. Let rest about 1 minute.

Cut in half.

Enjoy!

Philadelphia Roll

Things Needed

for 4 servings

2 cups sushi rice(460 g)

¼ cup seasoned rice vinegar(60 mL)

4 half sheets sushi grade nori

4 oz smoked salmon(115 g)

4 oz cream cheese(115 g), cut into matchsticks

1 small cucumber, cut into matchsticks

Method

Season the sushi rice with the rice vinegar, fanning and stirring until room temperature.

On the rolling mat place one sheet of nori with the rough side facing upwards.

Wet your hands and grab a handful of rice and place it on the nori. Spread the rice evenly throughout the nori without smushing the rice down.

Arrange, in a horizontal row 1 inch (2 cm) from the bottom, smoked salmon, cream cheese, and cucumber.

Grabbing both nori and the mat, roll the mat over the filling so the extra space at the bottom touches the other side, squeezing down to make a nice tight roll. Squeeze down along the way to keep the roll from holding its shape.

Transfer the roll onto a cutting board. Rub a knife on a damp paper towel before slicing the roll into six equal portions.

Enjoy!

Hearty Roasted Veggie Salad

Things Needed

for 4 servings

3 beets

1 cup olive oil(240 mL), divided

1 ½ teaspoons salt, divided

1 red onion, cut into wedges

4 carrots, peeled and chopped

2 parsnips, peeled, chopped

1 sweet potato, peeled, chopped

¾ teaspoon pepper, divided

2 tablespoons balsamic vinegar

1 tablespoon lemon juice

1 tablespoon dijon mustard

½ teaspoon garlic powder

3 tablespoons fresh parsley, chopped

6 cups mixed greens(600 g)

1 cup walnuts(100 g), chopped

½ cup crumbled feta cheese(55 g)

Method

Preheat oven to 425°F (220°C).

On a cutting board, cut the root end of the beet so it lays flat on the surface. Place the beet on a piece of aluminum foil. Drizzle with 1 tablespoon of olive oil and season with ¼ teaspoon salt. Wrap the foil around the beet and pinch the top of the foil together until the beet is sealed in. Repeat with the other 2 beets.

On a sheet pan, place the onions, carrots, parsnips, and sweet potato.

Drizzle with 3 tablespoons olive oil and season with ½ teaspoon pepper and ½ teaspoon salt. Toss the the vegetables until coated and spread them evenly in the pan.

Create 3 circular spaces for the beets. Place the 3 beets on the pan.

Bake for 1 hour until with vegetables begin to crisp and caramelize.

In a large bowl, add ½ cup (120 ml) of olive oil, balsamic vinegar, lemon juice, Dijon mustard, and garlic powder, and whisk until emulsified. Add the parsley and season with salt and pepper, stirring to combine.

Add the mixed greens, roasted vegetables, and the beets to the bowl with the vinaigrette and toss until evenly incorporated.

Serve with walnuts and feta.

Enjoy!

Shrimp & Avocado Tostadas

Things Needed

for 6 tostadas

6 corn tortillas

olive oil, to taste

1 lb shrimp(455 g), peeled and deveined

1 cup english cucumber(135 g), diced

1 cup tomato(200 g), diced

1 avocado, diced

1 cup red onion(150 g), diced

1 lemon, juiced

1 lime, juiced

1 tablespoon fresh cilantro, chopped

salt, to taste

1 serrano pepper, finely chopped, optional

Method

Preheat oven to 425°F (220°C).

Lay the corn tortillas on a parchment paper-lined baking sheet and lightly brush both sides with olive oil.

Bake the tortillas for 5 minutes and then flip them over continue baking another 5 minutes. The tostadas should be brown and crispy. Set the pan aside to cool.

Roughly chop the shrimp and transfer to a bowl.

Add the cucumber, tomato, avocado, red onion, lemon juice, lime juice, cilantro, salt, and serrano chile (optional), and stir to combine.

Marinate for 10-15 minutes.

Spoon the shrimp mixture onto the tostadas.

Enjoy!

Homemade Honey Mustard Chicken Salad

Things Needed

for 1 serving

DRESSING

1 tablespoon mustard

1 tablespoon honey

½ tablespoon olive oil

1 squeeze lemon juice

¼ teaspoon salt

¼ teaspoon pepper

¼ teaspoon garlic powder

SALAD

2 cups romaine lettuce(140 g), chopped

¼ cup red onion(35 g), sliced

¼ cup cherry tomato(50 g), halved

¼ cup avocado(35 g), diced

1 rotisserie chicken breast, sliced

1 egg, hard boiled and sliced

Method

In a small bowl, add mustard, honey, olive oil, lemon juice, salt, pepper, and garlic powder. Stir until combined.

In a large bowl, add lettuce, onion, tomatoes, avocado, and chicken.

Drizzle with honey mustard dressing and toss until evenly coated.

Serve with hard-boiled egg.

Enjoy!

WHOLESOME RECIPES FOR DINNER

Sweet Potato And Black Bean Burritos

Things Needed

for 3 servings

2 medium sweet potatoes, peeled and cubed

olive oil, to taste

½ teaspoon smoked paprika

½ teaspoon garlic powder

kosher salt, to taste

freshly ground black pepper, to taste

½ medium yellow onion, diced

1 jalapeño, seeded and diced

1 clove garlic, minced

1 teaspoon chili powder

½ teaspoon ground cumin

cayenne pepper, to taste

15 oz black beans(425 g), drained and rinsed

¾ cup corn(130 g)

3 large flour tortillas

FOR SERVING

chopped lettuce

diced tomato

shredded vegan cheddar cheese

guacamole

Method

Preheat the oven to 400°F (200°C).

Add the sweet potatoes to a baking sheet with a drizzle of olive oil, the paprika, garlic powder, salt, and black pepper. Toss until well-coated.

Bake for 20 minutes, flipping halfway through, until the sweet potato is tender.

Heat a drizzle of olive oil in a large saucepan over medium heat. Once the oil begins to shimmer, add the onion and cook for 3-4 minutes, until semi-translucent. Add the jalapeño, garlic, chili powder, cumin, and cayenne pepper and cook for 2-3 minutes, until the spices are fragrant. Add the black beans and corn, season with salt and pepper, and cook until warmed through, 3-4 more minutes.

To assemble a burrito, add one-third of the bean and corn mixture, one-third of the roasted sweet potatoes, some lettuce, tomatoes, vegan cheese, and guacamole to the center of a tortilla. Fold in the sides and roll up, keeping the filling tucked in place. Repeat with the remaining **Things Needed**. Cut in half and serve.

Enjoy!

One-pan Chicken Sausage & Veggies

Things Needed

for 4 servings

1 zucchini, sliced

1 yellow squash, sliced

1 tablespoon olive oil

¼ teaspoon salt

¼ teaspoon pepper

¼ teaspoon garlic powder

4 chicken sausages, fully cooked, sliced

4 cups wild rice(920 g), cooked, to serve

Method

Preheat the oven to 400°F (200°C).

Place the squash and zucchini on a baking sheet. Evenly coat with olive oil, salt, pepper, and garlic powder.

Push the squash and zucchini to the sides and place the chicken sausage in the middle.

Bake for 15 minutes, or until the zucchini and squash are tender.

Serve with wild rice. Eat immediately or refrigerate in airtight container up to 3-4 days.

Enjoy!

Steak Fajita Quesadillas

Things Needed

for 4 servings

1 lb skirt steak(455 g)

2 tablespoons olive oil

salt, to taste

pepper, to taste

1 teaspoon chili powder

1 teaspoon cumin

1 onion, sliced

4 cloves garlic, sliced

3 bell peppers, sliced

1 jalapeño pepper, sliced

1 tablespoon butter

4 large tortillas

2 cups mexican blend cheese(200 g)

guacamole

sour cream

salsa

Method

Season skirt steak with olive oil, salt, pepper, chili powder, and cumin.

Cook on high heat for roughly 3 minutes each side, for medium-rare.

Let the steak rest for 10 minutes.

While the steak is resting, sauté onion and garlic until slightly translucent. Add bell peppers, jalapeño, salt, and pepper, cook slightly.

Slice the steak into strips.

Mix the steak into the pepper mix. Remove from heat and set aside.

In a clean pan, melt butter. Lay the tortilla on the buttered pan, add cheese, fajita mixture, more cheese, then top with another tortilla and pat it down.

Flip the quesadilla over and cook the other side until it's golden.

Remove from pan and cut into quarters or eighths. Repeat these steps with the remaining tortillas.

Serve immediately with sour cream, salsa, and guacamole.

Enjoy!

Easy Chicken Paprikash

Things Needed

for 2 servings

1 tablespoon oil

1 tablespoon garlic

2 chicken thighs, cut into bite-sized pieces

1 teaspoon salt

½ teaspoon pepper

1 cup onion(150 g), chopped

½ cup bell pepper(50 g), chopped

2 tablespoons sweet paprika

¼ teaspoon chili flakes

½ cup chicken broth(120 mL)

15 oz crushed tomato(425 g), 1 can

½ cup sour cream(115 g)

1 tablespoon flour

Method

Heat oil over medium, add garlic, chicken, salt and pepper. Stir and cook until the chicken has some color.

Add the onion and bell pepper, cook until onions have slightly softened.

Add the sweet paprika, chili flakes, chicken broth and crushed tomatoes. Simmer covered for 40 minutes.

Take a ladle of the sauce and add to sour cream in a separate bowl. Mix until well combined. Add flour to the mix and stir.

Once it is well combined, add the mix to the pot. Stir in the mix, cover and simmer for an additional 5 minutes or until it has thickened.

Serve with pasta, rice or potatoes.

Enjoy!

Beef & Bean Burritos

Things Needed

for 6 burritos

1 lb ground beef(455 g)

2 tablespoons taco seasoning

6 flour tortillas

16 oz refried bean(455 g), 1 can

1 cup shredded mexican cheese blend(100 g)

Method

Add ground beef to a large skillet over high heat and sprinkle with taco seasoning. Cook, breaking up the meat, until browned. Drain the fat and set aside to cool.

Assemble the burritos by microwaving the flour tortilla for 20 seconds, and begin to layer burrito starting with refried beans, followed by the cooked beef and cheese.

Fold in the left and right sides of the tortilla and roll it up from the bottom, tucking the bottom edge under the filling. Wrap in parchment paper and label. Freeze up to 1 month.

To reheat from frozen, wrap the burrito in a damp paper towel and microwave for 2-3 minutes, flipping halfway or until the center is hot. Let stand 1 minute before eating.

Enjoy!

One-Pan Moroccan Chicken

Things Needed

for 2 servings

2 boneless, skinless chicken breasts

ground black pepper, to taste

ground cumin, to taste

1 teaspoon neutral oil

½ onion, sliced

½ can cherry tomatoes

⅖ cup water(100 mL)

½ can chickpeas, drained and rinsed

1 tablespoon harissa paste

1 teaspoon honey

1 courgette, sliced

Method

Season the chicken with pepper and cumin.

Heat the oil in a large, high-walled pan over medium-low heat. Add the chicken and onion and cook for 3-4 minutes, stirring and turning occasionally.

Add the cherry tomatoes, water, chickpeas, harissa, honey, and courgette. Simmer for 15 minutes, stirring occasionally, until the sauce thickens.

Enjoy!

Protein-Packed Chili

Things Needed

for 8 servings

1 tablespoon oil

8 cloves garlic, minced

1 onion, chopped

1 red bell pepper, chopped

1 jalapeño, chopped, seeded

1 teaspoon salt, to taste

¼ teaspoon pepper, to taste

1 tablespoon cayenne pepper

4 tablespoons chili powder

1 tablespoon cumin

4 tomatoes, cubed

28 oz crushed tomato(795 g), 1 can

4 cups vegetable broth(960 mL)

2 cups water(480 mL)

1 ½ cups quinoa(255 g), rinsed

1 cup red kidney bean(175 g), drained

1 cup pinto bean(175 g), drained

1 cup black beans(170 g), drained

1 cup corn(175 g), fresh or frozen

1 tablespoon lime juice

1 teaspoon dried oregano

1 tablespoon fresh cilantro

avocado, for garnish

Method

In a large pot, over medium heat, combine oil, garlic, onion, pepper, jalapeño, salt, pepper, cayenne pepper, chili powder, and cumin. Sauté until onion is translucent, 5-6 minutes.

Add tomatoes, crushed tomatoes, vegetable broth, water, quinoa, kidney beans, pinto beans, and black beans. Bring to a boil.

Cover and reduce to a simmer for 25-30 minutes.

Add corn, lime juice, oregano, and cilantro, cover again and simmer for 5 minutes.

Allow to cool 2 minutes. Serve topped with avocado and cilantro.

Enjoy!

Slow Cooker Chicken Fajita Bowls

Things Needed

for 8 servings

1 red bell pepper, sliced

1 yellow bell pepper, sliced

1 green bell pepper, sliced

1 yellow onion, sliced

2 lb chicken breast(910 g), sliced in half

2 tablespoons taco seasoning

salt, to taste

pepper, to taste

4 garlics, minced

1 lime, juiced

1 can diced tomato, drained

4 cups brown rice(920 g), cooked

GARNISH

sour cream

guacamole

fresh cilantro

shredded cheese

Method

In a slow cooker, place half of the bell peppers and onion.

Lay on the chicken, and coat both sides with taco seasoning, salt, and pepper.

Sprinkle on garlic, half of the lime juice, and diced tomatoes. Cover with remaining peppers, onion, and lime juice.

Cover and cook on high for 3 hours.

Remove chicken from the slow cooker, shred, and return to slow cooker.

Cover until heated through.

Serve over brown rice with sour cream, guacamole, shredded cheese and cilantro.

Enjoy!

Chickpea Sweet Potato Stew

Things Needed

for 4 servings

2 tablespoons refined coconut oil

1 small onion, diced

3 cloves garlic, minced

1 teaspoon ginger, minced

1 tablespoon sweet paprika

½ teaspoon cumin

¼ teaspoon dried coriander

⅛ teaspoon cayenne

15 oz canned chickpeas(425 g), drained and rinsed

2 cups peeled and diced sweet potatoes(400 g)

15 oz canned fire-roasted crushed tomatoes(425 g)

3 cups vegetable broth(720 mL)

5 oz fresh spinach(140 g)

Method

In large pot or Dutch oven, heat the coconut oil over medium heat. Once the oil begins to shimmer, add the onion and cook for 4-5 minutes, or until the onion is semi-translucent.

Add the garlic and ginger, and cook for 2-3 more minutes, until fragrant. Then add the sweet paprika, cumin, coriander, and cayenne and cook for 2 more minutes, until fragrant.

Add the chickpeas, sweet potatoes, crushed tomatoes, and vegetable broth, and bring to a boil. Reduce the heat to medium-low and simmer for 15-20 minutes, or until the sweet potatoes are tender.

Add the spinach and stir until wilted.

Serve immediately.

Enjoy!

Lemon Pepper Chicken and Rice

Things Needed

for 4 servings

3 tablespoons lemon pepper

1 tablespoon paprika

2 cloves garlic, minced

1 tablespoon olive oil

2 lb chicken thighs with skin(910 g)

4 tablespoons butter

1 yellow onion, diced

1 ½ cups arborio rice(300 g)

¼ cup white wine(60 mL)

4 cups chicken broth(960 mL)

1 ½ cups milk(360 mL)

pepper, to taste

1 cup parmesan cheese(100 g)

¼ cup fresh parsley(10 g), optional

Method

Combine lemon pepper, paprika, and 2 cloves of minced garlic in a small bowl.

In a large oven-proof pot, heat olive oil on medium heat. Season both sides of the chicken and place in the pot skin side down. Cook for three minutes, turn the heat up to medium high and cook for an additional two minutes (or until browned). Turn the chicken over and cook for another 3-4 minutes. Remove chicken from the pot and set aside. (Don't worry! It will finish cooking when you put it in the oven.)

With a paper towel, carefully wipe out excess fat, leaving the seasoning.

Preheat your oven to 350°F (175°C).

On medium high, melt two Tbsp. of butter in the pot and add the diced onions and the rest of the minced garlic. Cook until onions are translucent (1-2 minutes).

Add the rice and stir until it becomes translucent (1-2 minutes).

Pour in the white wine and let it cook until most of the wine has evaporated (about two minutes).

Add the chicken broth, one cup of milk, and a dash of pepper and stir. Bring it to a simmer.

Place the chicken back into the pot. Cover with a lid or foil and bake for 30 minutes (remove lid after 20 minutes).

Remove the chicken from the pot and broil on high for 2-3 minutes or until the skin has nicely browned.

Add the other two Tbsp. butter, parmesan, ½ cup (118 ml) of milk and parsley to the rice. Stir until well combined. Return the chicken on top of the rice.

Enjoy!

Garlic Mashed Sweet Potatoes

Things Needed

for 4 servings

4 sweet potatoes

2 tablespoons butter(30 g)

¼ cup heavy cream(60 mL)

3 cloves garlic, minced

1 teaspoon salt

1 teaspoon pepper

Method

Add potatoes to a large pot of salted water. Place over medium/high heat and bring to a boil. Cook until fork tender, about 15-20 minutes.

Drain, peel, and mash potatoes until they reach a smooth consistency.

Add remaining **Things Needed** to mash and mix to incorporate.

Enjoy!

Chicken Tortilla Bowl Soup

Things Needed

for 8 servings

1 onion, diced

1 jalapeño, diced

3 cloves garlic, chopped

3 chicken breasts

1 can black beans, drained

1 can corn, drained

1 can diced tomato

1 can red enchilada sauce

4 cups chicken stock(945 mL)

½ teaspoon dried oregano

½ teaspoon ground pepper

1 teaspoon cumin

1 teaspoon salt

1 pack large flour tortilla

vegetable oil, for frying

TOPPINGS (OPTIONAL)

fresh cilantro

monterey jack cheese

lime, wedged

avocado, sliced

Method

Place diced onion, jalapeno and garlic in the bottom of a slow cooker.

Place the chicken breasts on top of the veggies.

Add all canned **Things Needed** and seasonings to the chicken in the slow cooker. Top with the chicken stock.

Set slow cooker to high and cook for 3 hours.

Fill a large pot ⅔ full with vegetable oil and heat until it reaches 350°F (180°C).

Carefully place the tortilla on top of the oil and gently press the tortilla down with a ladle. Fry tortilla until golden brown. Drain on a cooling rack.

When soup is done, remove chicken and dice it on a cutting board. Return diced chicken to the soup.

Place fried tortilla bowl in a soup bowl and fill it with the soup.

Top it off with cheese, avocado, cilantro and garnish with a lime wedge.

Enjoy!!

Chili Cheese Casserole

Things Needed

for 6 servings

15 oz bean chili(425 g), 1 can

8 oz tomato sauce(225 g), 1 can

8 tortillas

2 cups shredded cheddar cheese(200 g)

Method

In a bowl, add the chili and tomato sauce and stir to combine.

Add a layer of the chili mixture to the bottom of a 9x9-inch (23x23-cm) baking pan. Top with a layer of tortillas, a layer of chili, and sprinkle with cheese.

Repeat until all **Things Needed** are used, making sure the top layer is cheese.

Cover and refrigerate for at least 3 hours, up to overnight.

Preheat oven to 350°F (180°C).

Remove the casserole from the refrigerator and let sit for 10 minutes on your counter.

Poke three toothpicks in the casserole, and cover with tin foil, so that the foil doesn't touch the cheese layer.

Bake for 30-40 minutes, or until cheese is melted.

Cut and serve.

Enjoy!

French Pepper Steak (Steak Au Poivre)

Things Needed

for 2 servings

2 tablespoons whole black peppercorns

14 oz new york strip steak(400 g), or other good-quality steak

2 teaspoons kosher salt

1 tablespoon vegetable oil

2 tablespoons unsalted butter, divided

⅓ cup brandy or cognac(80 mL)

1 cup cream(240 mL)

1 tablespoon dijon mustard

Method

Wrap the peppercorns in a lint-free kitchen towel, then smash with the bottom of a skillet until coarsely crushed.

Liberally season the steak on all sides with the salt and crushed peppercorns, using your hands to press the seasoning into the meat to create an even coating.

Heat the vegetable oil and 1 tablespoon of butter in a large skillet over medium-high heat until just smoking. Add the steak to the pan and sear for 4 minutes. Flip and sear the other side for another 4 minutes, for medium-rare. If steak has a fat-cap on its side, be sure to sear it as well for 30–60 seconds. Once cooked to desired doneness, transfer the steak to a cutting board to rest.

Reduce the heat to medium and add the brandy to the skillet. Allow the brandy to cook down for about 1 minute while using a whisk to scrape up any browned bits in the bottom of the pan. Once the brandy has reduced by half, add the cream, mustard, and remaining tablespoon of butter and continue to cook until the mixture begins to reduce and thicken, 5-7 minutes. The sauce should have a rich consistency and coat the back of a spoon.

Slice the steak into ½-inch (1½-cm) pieces. Pour the sauce over the top and serve.

Enjoy!

Slow-Cooker Pot Roast

Things Needed

for 6 servings

1 ½ lb baby potato(680 g), red and/or yellow

8 small carrots, snapped in half

12 pearl onions, peeled, with ends cut off

3 ½ lb beef chuck roast(1 ½ kg)

salt, to taste

pepper, to taste

1 tablespoon cornstarch

2 tablespoons water

2 tablespoons worcestershire sauce

2 sprigs fresh rosemary

2 sprigs fresh thyme

1 baguette, cut into 5-inch (13 cm) pieces, optional

Method

In a slow cooker, add the potatoes, carrots, and onions to make a base for the meat.

Lay the chuck roast on top of the veggies and season with salt and pepper on both sides.

Wash your hands, because mess.

Mix cornstarch and water until well combined and pour close to the edge so it gets down to the veggies.

Pour Worcestershire sauce directly on top of the meat.

Cover with the slow-cooker lid and cook on high for 5 hours.

Place the rosemary and thyme sprigs on top of the meat and cook for 1 more hour.

Remove rosemary and thyme.

Using a fork, shred the meat and serve by itself with the veggies, or on top of bread for a sandwich! The juices from the bottom of the slow cooker make for an AMAZING dipping sauce!

Enjoy!

WHOLESOME RECIPES FOR SNACKS

Bacon Green Bean Twists

Things Needed

for 2 servings

1 sheet puff pastry

½ lb bacon(225 g)

½ lb green beans(225 g), trimmed

1 egg, beaten

salt, to taste

pepper, to taste

Method

Preheat the oven to 400°F (200°C).

Cut one sheet of puff pastry into long ½ inch (1 ¼ cm) wide strips and set aside.

Cut strips of bacon in half lengthwise and set aside.

Take a trimmed green bean and carefully wrap it with bacon and the puff pastry to completely cover the bean.

Place the tightly wrapped beans on a parchment paper-lined sheet pan. Brush the wrapped beans with the egg wash, and season with salt and pepper.

Bake in the oven for 20 minutes, or until bacon is crispy and the puff pastry is golden brown.

Serve the twists warm or at room temperature.

Enjoy!

Monkey Bread Brie Fondue

Things Needed

for 6 servings

1 tablespoon unsalted butter

1 medium white onion, thinly sliced

26 oz pizza dough(735 g)

½ cup bacon(110 g), chopped

4 tablespoons unsalted butter, 1/2 stick, melted

8 oz brie cheese(225 g), 1 wheel

1 fresh chive, chopped, for garnish

broccoli floret, steamed, for serving

1.5 lb baby potato(680 g), boiled, halved, for serving

mushroom, sauteed, for serving

Method

Preheat the oven to 400°F (200°C). Prepare a 9-inch (22 cm) round cake pan with a 3½- inch (8 cm) ramekin in the center and set nearby.

Melt the butter in a large pan over medium-low heat. Add the onion and sauté until caramelized, stirring occasionally for about 15 minutes. Remove the pan from the heat.

Take a golf ball-sized piece of pizza dough and flatten it out with your fingers. Stuff the dough with about a teaspoon of caramelized onions and cooked bacon. Close the dough ball by pinching at the seam and roll into a ball in your hands. Repeat with the remaining dough and fillings.

Dip each stuffed ball in the melted butter. Place the stuffed balls in the prepared cake pan, stacking them around the ramekin.

Bake for 30 minutes, or until golden brown. Remove from the oven and reduce the oven temperature to 350°F (180°C). Remove the ramekin with tongs (it will be hot!).

Place the wheel of brie in the center. Return the pan to the oven for 10 minutes more, or until the brie is soft.

Brush the monkey bread with more melted butter and sprinkle the bread and cheese with chives. Serve with vegetables like broccoli, potatoes, and mushrooms for dipping.

Enjoy!

Easy Pantry Hummus

Things Needed

for 4 servings

15 oz garbanzo beans(425 g)

½ teaspoon kosher salt

½ teaspoon ground cumin

1 clove garlic, minced

2 tablespoons lemon juice

¼ cup water(60 mL)

2 tablespoons olive oil, plus more for garnish

paprika, for garnish

chips, crackers, and/or vegetable, for serving

Method

Drain the garbanzo beans, reserving the liquid. Rinse the garbanzos.

Add the garbanzo beans to a blender, along with the salt, cumin, and garlic. Blend on medium speed. While the blender is running, pour in the lemon juice, water, and olive oil. Continue blending until the hummus is smooth.

Transfer the hummus to a serving dish and use a spoon to smooth the top. Top with a drizzle of olive oil and a sprinkle of paprika.

Cover and chill until ready to serve. Serve with your choice of crackers, chips, or vegetables.

Enjoy!

Sour Cream And Onion Mozzarella Sticks

Things Needed

for 6 sticks

3 cups sour cream and onion-flavoured crisps(100 g), crushed

2 tablespoons plain flour

1 teaspoon paprika

1 teaspoon onion salt

2 teaspoons dried chive, plus more for serving

2 eggs

6 sticks string cheese

oil, for frying

Method

Crush the crisps in a zip top bag with a rolling pin, or just blend them for a few seconds in a food processor. Add to a small bowl and set aside.

In another small bowl, combine flour, paprika, onion salt, and chives.

In one more separate bowl, beat 2 eggs.

Coat the string cheese in flour first, then egg, then crisps. Then go back into the egg, and again in the crisps for an extra crispy breading.

Heat a skillet with a bit of oil in the bottom and cook mozzarella sticks for 3 to 5 minutes, turning occasionally to brown all sides.

Sprinkle a pinch of salt and with more dried chives, and serve with sour cream dip!

Enjoy!

Sopaipillas

Things Needed

for 12 sopaipillas

DOUGH

2 cups all purpose flour(250 g), plus more for dusting

2 teaspoons granulated sugar

1 ½ teaspoons vegetable oil, plus more for frying

1 teaspoon baking powder

1 teaspoon kosher salt

¼ cup whole milk(60 mL)

½ cup warm water(120 mL)

CHOCOLATE DIPPING SAUCE

¼ cup dark chocolate chips(45 g)

¼ cup semi-sweet chocolate chips(45 g)

1 teaspoon coconut oil

½ teaspoon ancho chile powder

½ teaspoon cinnamon

3 tablespoons heavy cream, warmed

½ teaspoon vanilla extract

ASSEMBLY

¼ cup honey(85 g)

¼ cup powdered sugar(30 g)

Method

Make the dough: In a large bowl, whisk together the flour, sugar, vegetable oil, baking powder, and salt. Add the milk and warm water and stir with a rubber spatula until a sticky dough forms.

Turn the dough out onto a lightly floured surface and knead for 2-3 minutes, until no longer sticky.

Place the dough on a plate or baking sheet and cover with a damp cloth. Let rest for 15 minutes.

Divide the dough into 3 equal balls, cover again with damp cloth, and let rest for 30-60 minutes.

Make the chocolate dipping sauce: Add the dark and milk chocolate and coconut oil to a medium microwave-safe bowl. Microwave in 30-second increments, stirring in between, until the chocolate is melted. Stir in the ancho chile powder and cinnamon. Whisk in the warm cream, 1 tablespoon at a time, until a thin dipping sauce consistency is reached. Stir in the vanilla. Set aside.

Fill a Dutch oven or large pot fitted with a deep fry thermometer with about 3 inches (7 cm) of vegetable oil. Heat the oil until it reaches 400°F (200°C).

While the oil is heating, shape the sopaipillas: On a lightly floured surface, roll out 1 of the 3 dough balls to a 8-inch (20 cm) square. Cut into 4 4-inch (10 cm) squares, discarding any extra trimmed dough. Place the squares on a baking sheet and cover with a damp towel. Repeat with the remaining dough.

Line a baking sheet with paper towels and set near the pot of oil.

Gently transfer one square of dough into the hot oil as a tester--it should float to the surface within a few seconds. As soon as the dough floats, flip it over immediately. Keep turning the dough every 5 seconds or so, until it puffs up like a pillow and turns light golden brown, about 1 minute. Remove from the oil and drain on the prepared baking sheet. Repeat with the remaining dough squares, frying 2-4 at a time, or however many will fit without crowding the pot.

Drizzle half of the sopaipillas with the honey and dust with the powdered sugar. Serve the other half with chocolate dipping sauce. Serve immediately.

Enjoy!

Garlic And Herb Hummus

Things Needed

for 6 servings

15 oz garbanzo beans(425 g), 1 can

2 cloves garlic

3 tablespoons tahini

1 lemon, juiced

2 tablespoons olive oil, more to garnish

salt, to taste

pine nut, to garnish

1 ½ tablespoons fresh parsley

2 tablespoons water

pita chip, to serve

Method

Boil the garbanzo beans until the skins come off.
Remove the skins, drain.

Combine all **Things Needed** in a food processor.

Blend until smooth adding small amounts of oil
and water until desired consistency is achieved.

Add more lemon or tahini if needed.

Garnish with pine nuts and more oil!

Eat with fresh vegetables or pita chips.

Enjoy!

Baked Artichoke Bites

Things Needed

for 4 servings

1 cup panko bread crumbs(50 g)

½ cup vegetarian parmesan cheese(60 g)

½ cup salted butter(125 mL), 1 stick, melted

15 oz canned artichoke heart(425 g), 2 cans, drained, rinsed, and patted dry

fresh parsley, chopped, for serving

GARLIC AIOLI

½ cup mayonnaise(115 g)

2 tablespoons olive oil

1 teaspoon garlic, minced

1 tablespoon lemon juice

¼ teaspoon salt

¼ cup fresh parsley(10 g), chopped

Method

Preheat the oven to 400°F (200°C). Line a baking sheet with parchment paper and set a wire rack inside.

Drain and rinse the artichokes. Pat them dry.

In a medium bowl, combine the bread crumbs and vegetarian Parmesan cheese.

Dip the artichoke hearts in the melted butter, making sure they are evenly coated. Then coat well with the bread crumb mixture.

Place the artichoke bites on the wire rack.

Bake for 15 minutes, then reduce the oven temperature to 350°F (175°C), flip the artichokes, and bake for 15 minutes more, until the artichoke hearts are warmed through and the bread crumb mixture is toasted.

Meanwhile, make the garlic aioli. In a small bowl, combine the mayonnaise, olive oil, garlic, lemon juice, salt, and parsley. Stir to combine.

Sprinkle the artichoke bites with parsley before serving with aioli alongside.

Enjoy!

Cream Cheese-Stuffed Bagel Bites

Things Needed

for 10 bites

1 cup water(240 mL), warm, plus 2 tbsp

1 teaspoon instant dry yeast

1 tablespoon malt syrup

3 ½ cups bread flour(420 g)

2 teaspoons salt

POACHING LIQUID THINGS NEEDED

2 qt water(2 L)

2 teaspoons salt

1 tablespoon baking soda

2 tablespoons malt syrup

egg wash, as needed

BAGEL TOPPING AND FILLING

onion, to taste

poppy seed, to taste

sesame seed, to taste

garlic, to taste

cream cheese, frozen in 1 tbsp. balls to taste

Method

Start by activating the yeast. Add yeast and malt syrup to warm water, stir until dissolved. Once the yeast mix starts bubbling, you'll know the yeast is active.

Combine the dry **Things Needed** in a large mixing bowl. Add the activated yeast mix and form a loose dough in the bowl.

Turn dough out onto your surface and knead until everything comes together nicely. (If it's too dry, add more water a little bit at a time.) Transfer dough to an oiled bowl, cover and let the dough rest for 45 minutes.

While the dough is resting, prep your cream cheese. Freeze cream cheese into 1 tbsp. balls.

Punch down dough after 45 minutes, knead the dough a few times. Pull a handful of dough, form into a ball then flatten and wrap around a frozen cream cheese ball. Repeat with the rest of the dough. Place bagel balls on a parchment paper, cover and let it rest for 20 minutes.

While the bagel balls are resting, bring your poaching liquid **Things Needed** to a boil over medium heat.

Take the rested bagel balls and boil in the poaching liquid for 15-20 seconds. Remove and place on parchment paper.

Brush with egg wash and sprinkle desired bagel toppings.

Bake in 325°F (160°C) preheated oven for 20 - 30 minutes until top is golden brown.

Enjoy!

Buffalo Chicken Hand Pies

Things Needed

for 10 hand pies

2 cups rotisserie chicken(250 g), shredded

1 cup cream cheese(225 g), softened

1 cup Frank's® buffalo sauce(230 g)

½ cup shredded mozzarella cheese(50 g)

¼ cup red onion(35 g)

½ teaspoon fresh ground black pepper

1 teaspoon celery salt

2 square sheets pie dough

2 egg yolks, beaten

1 cup ranch dressing(235 g), for serving

Method

Preheat the oven to 400°F (200°C). Line 2 baking sheets with parchment paper.

In a medium bowl, combine the shredded chicken, cream cheese, buffalo sauce, mozzarella, red onion, black pepper, and celery salt. Mix until thoroughly combined.

Unroll the pie dough and cut out 4 circles from each sheet using a 3½-inch (8.75 cm) round cutter.

Re-roll and cut out as many circles as you can, about 10 total. Discard the dough scraps. Place the dough circles on the prepared baking sheets.

Fill each dough circle with 1 heaping tablespoon of the buffalo chicken filling. Fold in half to form a half-moon shape. Using a fork, press all along the outer edges to seal the dough together. Brush all over with the beaten egg yolks.

Bake for 12–15 minutes, turning halfway, until the pies are slightly puffed and golden,. Remove from oven and let cool slightly.

Serve the hand pies warm with ranch dressing alongside.

Enjoy!

Lemon Pepper Cauliflower Bites

Things Needed

for 2 servings

1 large head cauliflower

1 ½ tablespoons olive oil

salt, to taste

1 teaspoon fresh cracked pepper, to taste

Method

Preheat oven to 400°F (200°C).

Break the head of cauliflower into bite-sized florets.

In a large bowl, combine olive oil, salt and pepper.

Add the cauliflower and coat well.

Transfer cauliflower to an oiled, parchment-lined baking sheet and bake for 20 minutes.

Remove from oven and squeeze the juice of one lemon over the florets. Adding the lemon juice in the beginning prevents the cauliflower from getting soggy. Top with some more cracked pepper if you prefer.

Bake for another 10 minutes or until heated through.

Serve with aioli or your favorite dipping sauce.

Enjoy!

Tangy Tortilla Chips

Things Needed

for 4 servings

12 corn tortillas, 4 inch (10 cm) wide

¼ cup olive oil(60 mL)

2 tablespoons McCormick® Tangy Spice Blend, divided

2 teaspoons kosher salt, divided, plus more to taste

Method

Preheat oven to 350°F (180°C). Line 2 baking sheets with parchment paper.

Lightly brush the tortillas all over with olive oil. Sprinkle ¼ teaspoon of tangy spice blend evenly over each tortilla and season lightly with salt. Flip and repeat on the other sides.

Stack 4 tortillas on top of one another and cut into 6 equal triangles. Repeat with the remaining tortillas.

Spread the tortilla triangles in a single layer on the prepared baking sheets.

Bake the tortillas for 20–25 minutes, rotating halfway through, until golden brown and crispy. Remove from the oven and let cool. The chips will continue to crisp as they cool.

Enjoy!

Chicken And Waffles Nachos

Things Needed

for 8 servings

2 cups buttermilk(480 mL)

3 teaspoons black pepper, divided

1 teaspoon kosher salt, plus more to taste

4 boneless, skinless chicken thighs, cubed

1 ½ cups maple syrup(505 g)

2 tablespoons vinegar based hot sauce

2 cups canola oil(240 mL), for frying

1 ½ cups all purpose flour(185 g)

½ teaspoon chili powder

½ teaspoon paprika

½ teaspoon garlic powder

3 large eggs

14 frozen waffles, cut into quarters

3 oz shredded cheddar cheese(85 g)

½ cup sour cream(120 mL)

2 tablespoons scallions, chopped

Method

In a large bowl, combine the buttermilk, 1 teaspoon of salt, and 1 teaspoon of black pepper. Place the chicken in the buttermilk mixture and toss to coat, then cover and marinate in the refrigerator for 1-2 hours, up to overnight.

Make the spicy maple syrup: In a small saucepan over medium heat, combine the maple syrup and hot sauce. Bring to a simmer, then cook for about 5 minutes, or until fragrant. Remove the pan from the heat and let cool. Set aside until ready to serve, or store in an airtight container in the refrigerator for up to 1 month.

Heat the oil in a large heavy-bottomed pot until it reaches 325°F (170°C). Line 2 baking sheets with paper towels and set nearby.

Working in batches, fry the quartered waffles in the hot oil for about 30 seconds on each side, or until golden brown. Transfer to a paper towel-lined baking sheet and season with salt.

In a large bowl, combine the flour, remaining 2 teaspoons of black pepper, chili powder, paprika, and garlic powder. In a medium bowl, beat the eggs well.

Set a wire rack inside a baking sheet.

Remove the chicken from the refrigerator and, working in batches, coat the chicken in the flour mixture, then in the eggs, then in the flour again. Place on the wire rack.

Working in batches, fry the chicken in the hot oil for 2-3 minutes, or until golden brown on the outside. Season with additional salt if desired. Transfer to a paper towel-lined baking sheet to drain.

Turn the oven to broil.

Arrange the fried waffles on a baking sheet, overlapping slightly. Top with the chicken and cheddar cheese.

Broil for 1-2 minutes, or until the cheese is bubbling. Watch carefully so it does not burn.

Drizzle the nachos with ½ cup (120 ML) of the spicy maple syrup, dollop on the sour cream, and scatter the scallions over the top. Serve with the remaining spicy maple syrup alongside

Enjoy!

Rosemary Steak Bites

Things Needed

for 2 servings

1 lb sirloin steak(455 g), cut into 1 in pieces (2 1/2 cm)

1 teaspoon kosher salt, plus more to taste

½ teaspoon freshly ground black pepper, plus more to taste

8 sprigs fresh rosemary, bottom 4 inches (10 cm) of leaves removed

2 tablespoons extra virgin olive oil

4 cloves garlic, gently smashed

5 tablespoons unsalted butter, divided

1 cup red wine(240 mL), such as Cabernet Sauvignon

1 teaspoon granulated sugar

Method

Heat a 12-inch (5 cm) cast iron skillet over medium-high heat for at least 10 minutes.

Add the steak to a medium bowl and season with the salt and pepper, tossing to coat evenly.

Thread 2 pieces of steak onto each rosemary sprig, sliding up the stem until the steak meets the leaves. Using scissors, trim the bottom of the sprigs so each end is about ½ inch long.

Add the olive oil and garlic to the pan, stir, and let heat for about 1 minute.

Once the oil begins to smoke, add 1 tablespoon of butter and stir to distribute. Place the skewers in the pan. Sear, without moving, for about 2 minutes, until a nice brown crust forms on one side. Using tongs, carefully flip each skewer over and brown on the other side, about 2 minutes more. Once cooked to your desired doneness, remove the steak skewers from the skillet and set on a clean baking sheet to rest.

Without reducing the heat, carefully pour the wine into the skillet. Cook until reduced to ¼ cup, 5–10 minutes. Once reduced, remove the garlic from the pan and discard.

Add the sugar and remaining 4 tablespoons of butter to the red wine reduction and stir until combined, 1–2 minutes.

Garnish the steak skewers lightly with salt and pepper, then transfer to a serving platter and spoon the sauce on top.

Serve immediately.

Enjoy!

Coconut Broth Clams

Things Needed

for 4 servings

CLAMS

2 lb littleneck clams(910 g), or 1½ pounds manila clams, scrubbed

cold water, for soaking

3 tablespoons sea salt

GRILLED BREAD

1 sourdough baguette

olive oil, for brushing

sea salt, to taste

COCONUT BROTH

1 tablespoon coconut oil

½ medium red onion, thinly sliced

2 large stalks lemongrass

3 tablespoons minced fresh ginger

4 cloves garlic, minced

1 teaspoon red pepper flakes, or 2 minced Thai chiles

1 cup dry white wine(240 mL)

1 tablespoon brown sugar

1 tablespoon fish sauce, or low-sodium soy sauce

2 cups vegetable broth(480 mL), or chicken broth

13 oz full-fat coconut milk(370 mL)

FOR GARNISH

thinly sliced scallion

chopped fresh cilantro

Method

Pick through the clams and discard any that are open and do not close when firmly tapped–these clams are dead and should not be eaten. Add the rest to a colander.

Rinse and scrub the remaining live clams to remove any sand or barnacles from the shells.

Fill a bowl large enough to fit the colander with cold water and 3-4 tablespoons of salt for every 6 cups (1.5 liters) of water. Place the colander in the bowl of salt water and soak the clams for at least 1 hour, up to overnight, so they release any grit and sand. The colander allows the grit to fall to the bottom of the bowl. Live clams will filter the water while they push out any impurities in the process.

Transfer the clams in the colander to another large bowl of fresh water to desalt for 15-30 minutes.

Grill the bread: Slice the sourdough baguette into ½-inch (1 cm) pieces.

Brush each slice with olive oil and sprinkle with salt.

Toast the bread on a grill pan over medium-high heat until golden brown and crusty, about 2 minutes per side. Set aside.

Make the coconut broth: Melt the coconut oil in a wok or large pan over medium heat. Add the red onion and cook until it starts to become translucent, about 3 minutes.

Firmly tap the lemongrass stalks with a wooden spoon to bruise, which helps release their aroma and flavor during cooking. Trim the ends, then slice into approximately 4-inch (10 cm) pieces.

Add the lemongrass to the wok, along with the ginger, garlic, and red pepper flakes. Cook until fragrant, about 3 minutes.

Carefully pour in the white wine and stir to deglaze the pan. Bring to a simmer and cook until reduced by half, about 5 minutes.

Add the brown sugar, fish sauce, vegetable broth, and coconut milk. Bring to a boil.

Add the clams, return to a boil, and cook for 5-8 minutes, or until all of the clams are fully opened. If any clams remain closed, discard them.

Discard the lemongrass stalks and divide the clams and broth between serving bowls. Garnish with scallions and cilantro and serve with the grilled bread for dipping.

Enjoy!

Homemade Ricotta Ravioli

Things Needed

for 2 servings

8 cups whole milk(1.9 L)

2 tablespoons lemon juice

2 cloves garlic, minced

6 oz baby spinach(170 g)

salt, to taste

1 egg

1 cup water(235 mL)

1 packet wonton wrapper

Method

In a large saucepan, bring the milk to a boil. Add lemon juice, stir and let sit for about 30 seconds.

Remove the milk from the heat, let stand for about 15 minutes to curdle.

Place a strainer over a deep bowl. Line the strainer with a cheese cloth of a clean kitchen towel. Pour the milk into the kitchen towel and let strain for about 30 minutes.

Discard the liquid.

Sauté spinach and garlic.

In a medium bowl, combine the ricotta and spinach. Salt to taste. Add one beaten egg.

Spoon mixture in the center of a wonton wrapper.

Moisten the edges of the wrapper with water. Top with another wonton wrapper. Gently seal around the filling in the center and the edges.

Boil ravioli for two minutes.

Drain ravioli and serve with your choice of sauce.

Enjoy!

SECTION 8: IN SUMMARY

The Fiber Diet is not just a temporary eating plan but a sustainable lifestyle choice that offers a multitude of health benefits. From improving digestive health and aiding in weight management to reducing the risk of chronic diseases such as heart disease and type 2 diabetes, the importance of dietary fiber cannot be overstated. By incorporating a variety of fiber-rich foods into your daily diet, you can enhance your overall well-being and support your body's natural functions at every life stage.

Understanding the different types of fiber, their sources, and how they affect the body empowers you to make informed dietary choices. Whether you are a child, an adult, a senior, or a pregnant or nursing woman, tailoring your fiber intake to meet your specific needs can help optimize your health outcomes.

Practical strategies such as gradually increasing fiber intake, staying well-hydrated, and diversifying your food choices are essential for integrating fiber into your diet effectively. Additionally, navigating common challenges and making use of fiber supplements when necessary can further ensure that you meet your daily fiber requirements.

Ultimately, embracing the Fiber Diet means committing to a balanced and nutritious approach to eating that promotes long-term health and vitality. By making fiber a cornerstone of your diet,

you invest in a healthier future for yourself and
your loved ones.